Let us think about this Rubric Today

(A desk top guide for those following Mind Methods in Homoeopathy)

Complied By

A.R Veeraraghavan.

**Lakshmi Homoeo House,
390B, Senthangudi Chetti Streeet,
Mayiladuthurai, Pin: 609 001,
Tamil Nadu, India.**

Let us think about this Rubric Today

Complied by : A. R Veeraraghavan,

First Edition August 2018

Published by :

Lakshmi Homeo House,
390B, Senthangudi Chetti Streeet,
Mayiladuthurai, Pin: 609 001
Tamil Nadu, India.
Email: arveehomoe@gmail.com

Note:

Information given in this book are not intended to be taken as a replacement for medical advice. Any person with a condition requiring medical advice should consult a qualified Homoeopathic Practitioner.

PREFACE

I am very glad to present this book. It will become a great desk top guide to who are interested in Prescribing on Mind Methods.

Homoeopathy plays a vital role in the world of health for billions of patient and are getting cure completely.

In Homoeopathy we treat the patient, not disease. So "Individuation' is the most important towards a successful practice. For the so called Individuation of the patients, following the Mind Rubrics is very important tool.

Dr. Hahnamann said in Organon – Aphorism 211 : ...."the state of disposition of the patient often chiefly determine the selection of the homoeopathic remedy...."

Mental state of patients are right enough to individualize any patient. It has been proved worldwide that true image of an individual can be easily perceived from mental symptoms.

It is easy to interpret the patient individually with observing patient's speech, attitude, behavior, gestures made, life style, etc. Selection of similimum has become simple and fast process with the help of repertory. It becomes easy to recognize the patient with the help of rubrics of Mind section of the Repertory.

Homoeopathic Repertories serve a great tool to Understand the Patient Language. But each and every word uttered by the patient is not there in any Repertory. We have to convert the patients' language into Rubrics of the Repertories. For that purpose this book will be very useful.

This book is about the practical knowledge of converting the patients' language into the language of repertory with great accuracy in the short span time.

For those who are already practice the Mind Methods (Like ROH or PROMISALONE, etc., understand the importance of this book.

Many stalwarts in Homoeopathy made a clear path towards to practice Mind Methods alone successfully. Dr. H. L. Chithkara, Dr. M. L. Sehgal, Dr. J.N. Kanjilal, and more Stalwarts are our Most Respectable Gurus to give us a right path to get clear successes.

I have included so many cases of my own clinical practice for better understanding. This book will serve an important source of this field of Homoeopathy.

Have a nice reading experience...!

Suggestions are welcomed towards the improvements of the book.

Readers may send the suggestions to my e-mail given below.
A.R. Veeraragavan,

Mayiladuthurai 609 001,

Tamil Nadu.

e-mail : arveehomeo@gmail.com

Let us think about this Rubrics Today..:

Let us think about this Rubric Today :1

ANSWERS, hardly

Only Remedy : IODIUM

(Hardly means : Scarcely./. Never)

Nearly three year ago, a girl of age 9 (Class IV Student) was brought to me for his complaints of severe stomach pain, ulceration in mouth and loss of appetite, by her mother. Allopathic treatments taken for the past few months did not give any relief.

Also she was very dull in her activities as well as her studies.

I asked her many questions. But she stared at her mother, not answered even a single question.

I asked her mother to stay in the waiting hall. Her mother tried to leave her, by that time also she just pulled her finger, not saying anything.

Her Mother went away my cabin.

I asked some questions about her school day functions, sports activities like to maintain pleasing situation.

But she sat and just saw the things in front of her in my table.

Even after ten minutes, she did not utter even a single word.

I took the rubrics,

1. ANSWERS, Hardly

And verified With the Rubric TIMIDITY, Bashful.

Iodium 30 was Prescribed.

After few days her physical problems solved.

After a month of Iodium 30, Her mother reported, that her nature also changed....Now she is somewhat active, and she got good marks in her studies.

Only **OIDIUM** 30. Only one dose, No other potencies, No other remedies...!

Now (Jan.2018) she is studying in Class VII, she is well in her studies.!

<u>*Let us think about this Rubric Today : 2*</u>

ANGER, Understood when not,

Remedies ; Bufo, laur, calc-s.

A short case :

It was about ten years back.

One male patient of age about 30, came for treatment for noise in his ears. He put some cotton in his both ears. When taking case I came to know that he had some sexual problems like premature ejaculations.

Due to his problems in his ear, he was unable to understand my questions.

I repeatedly questioned about his nature. He got angry when I talked to him loudly. (Actually I was likely to get anger..!)

After a long search I found the above beautiful Rubric.   On the basis of this entry rubric and other symptoms I prescribed Bufo 200C.
Surprisingly (I was new at that stage) his problems are settled well.
Have a nice day...!

Let us think about this Rubric Today : 3

ANGER, Interruption, form

Long back (nearly six years) A Class X student was brought by his father.

He runs a Medical Shop in our home town. It is the one of the biggest Medical shop.

His son has been suffering from persistent headache for the past few years.

As his father knows mostly all Allopaths in the town, many Allopaths treated him. Even specialists in that field did not give any relief to him. Lot of scan, ex-rays, investigations had been made. But nothing was indentified.

He consulted an eye specialist....But there was no defective in his eyes.

Medicines administrated. But no permanent cure.

Now

Conversation with the Student (Patient)

Doctor :"What are your problems.....?

He smiled and said, "Headache...Sir..."

Doctor: "When do you suffer....."

Patient : "Daily..sir.....often..it comes...."

Doctor: "So what...?

Patient: " Sir, It won't allow me to study..."(little bit irritated tone)

Now his father interpreted, " He had got good rank in the school. After this episode (Headache) he weeps that he is not able to study…."

Doctor: "Is there any other problems…?

Patient: "Often coryza formed…"

Medicine was given in 30c potency and PL also given for 15 days. And informed to report after a week.

After a week his father reported, he is normal now and studying without any interference .

Even now (June 2018), I often sees his father with his smiling face….!

Remedy : NUX VOMICA

Rubrics Selected :

ANGER, Interruption, form

BUSINESS, incapacity for

SMILING

Let us think about this Rubric Today : 4

MIND:- BUSY-Weak, Busy and.

Only remedy : MOSCHUS

We can understand This Rubric by the following case :

A male 35yrs old , running a mess[hotel] in his house comes with complaints of weakness, having this complaints for the past 1 year.

But didn't take treatment so for[may be interpreted as indifference/or frivolous] . Now also he was brought by his cousin for treatment, when he came for a marriage;.

While asked to tell about his complaints , He said that he feels very weak as he has to work hard to maintain the hotel , There is paucity of workers[labor]

So he and his wife has to do everything, like washing plates, serving [dining] cooking etc.

He wakes at 5 in the morning has to work till night 11pm;Then feels exhausted ,this was his routine, When asked why he didn't consult any doctor so far.

He said that he was too busy .possible rubrics came for him

[indifference/frivolous; helplessness; delusion poor or wearisome]

But I searched in the repertory and found a rubric

MIND:- BUSY-WEAK;BUSY

The remedy   MOSCHUS which cleared his weakness.

(Thanks World Homoeopathic Community)

Let us think about this Rubric Today : 5

MIND, Bending , forward agg:

Remedies: caust, coloc, glon, hell.

 This is given in the MIND Chapter. So we cannot take the meaning directly. It may be interpreted. I have no clinical experience about this rubric. But when discussed we get more ideas.

This is my interpretation :

When will we bend forward?

May be when we want to get somebody's apologies.

May be in subordination position to somebody, etc.,

So when the patient is forced to do so, his symptoms are aggravated.

Patient versions :

1. "I will be very discomfort to lean in front of anybody for my necessaries".

Let us Think about this Rubric Today : 6

BUSINESS, incapacity of,

A leady school teacher age about 35, working in a govt. school came to our Homoeopathic free camp held once in Second Saturday of every month. She has severe itching all over the body. Small rashes also appeared when she scratches..

The Conversation :

D: "Please be seated....what is your problem...?

 P: "Itching..doctor....If I take English Medicine, it will sustain for some days...then it will starts....."

D: "Next.....?

P: "I am not able to do my daily routines sir..I become very tired...."

D: " So what....?

 P: " I am not able to do anything sir....? My son is studying Higher secondary second year (+2)...Nobody in my home to help me....."

D: "Is..it...?"

P: "Sir Please..... do anything to stop my itching....I came here with the faith of you..."

Sepia **30c** Potency was given....and PL for 30 days (up to next camp). After a month she came for the free camp. She smiled at me and told that she was 90% better...slight itching was coming some times....

Only PL was given for
one more moth. She became normal afterwards.

Rubrics taken :

Disturbed, averse being
Business, incapacity of
Praying
Helplessness feeling of..
Delusion, alone she is
Cares full of domestic affairs

After a month she came for the free camp. She smiled at me and told that she was 90% better...slight itching was coming some times....

Only PL was given from one more moth, she became normal.

Let us think about this Rubric Today : 7

CURIOUS, Training of the Physician, wants to know the :

Only Remedy : Phos.

Here the patient is asking about the Qualifications, Experience of the doctor.

Some may ask, "Sir, don't mistake me, I think….Homoeopathy doctors are not as much trained as Allopathy doctors in the field of Anatomy and Physiology…."

It may be considered Phos. Is also in the following rubric:

WATCHFULLNESS,

1. Children are on the look out for every gesture.

2. every moment in the vicinity of every moment of doctor, of ,

****

<u>***Let us think about this rubric Today : 8***</u>

Mind: Carries things to and again back,

(Rophin Murphy)

Only remedy : Mag. Phos

It may be explained by a case:

(A case by Dr. K. Danabalan, BHMS, Madurai)
Few years back one school going boy of age 7 was brought by his parents for his complaints of cough and wheezing from the age of tow. He used Rotahaler three times a day. Allopathic treatment did not give any cure.

They also had treatments from various Homoeopathic doctors without any relief.

During my case taking I had noticed one peculiar behavior of the boy : While I talked with his mother he did play with pen stand, paper weight, pen etc., in my table. He carried one thing into the corner of the room. Then he took it back in the table. Like the same way he did for all things. I asked about this to his parents. They also confirmed that he was doing the same thing in the home.

I referred the Rubric : Mind, carries things to and again back. – in Rophin Murphy.. I prescribed Mag. Phos. 200. His complaints completely vanished in 3 months duration.

<u>*Let us Think about this Rubric Today : 9*</u>

DISTRUBED, Averse to being

(Taken as not being disturbed or not giving disturbance to anybody)

I give a case to get better understanding...

A case :

02.04.2011

A lady of age 42, who is residing in my street, known already, came to me for the treatment of coryza, cough and vertigo after cough.

"Sir, whenever I thank about to come for treatment, I had thought that you might be busy. And so as to not give trouble to you I did not come ...Is there any disturbance sir...?" (##)

No..Nothing..you may come at any time for treatment...ok.. what are your problems...?

"I am suffering form severe cough...I had taken treatment form Dr.........(Very popular Allopath in my home town). But no relief. The medicines given by that doctor leads to cough. Now I have giddiness after the cough....and a feeling of little unconsciousness after cough...."

"For how many days ....?"

"For the past six months...we are constructing our house...so I have to be present in the site....the dust particles and cement...etc...also affects me...."

I took the following Rubrics :

1. Disturbed, averse being

2. Delusion, wrong has suffered.

3. Delusion, Injured by his surroundings.

A dose of Naja 30 was prescribed.

Her problems settled beautifully.

After a month she brought her husband for treatment.

Note: (##) May be taken as : Anguish, for others.....(about doctor also!)

Let us think about this Rubric Today : 10

DELUSION, Blood is not circulates well,

Only Remedy : Atropinum Purum.

Following are the Patient's Versions :

1. I feel in my body the blood is not circulated well, that is why I have this   kind of pain all over the body.....(Direct Version).

2.   After this govt. is formed, money rotation is not well. So I face some financial crises.

3. Nowadays flow of money is not enough for me to face day to day needs.

(Interpreted: Money is as necessary as blood for survival !)

Let us think about this Rubric Today : 11

DELUSION, Paralyzed being, (he is)

Patient Versions :

1. " I need other's help even to wear my shirt..."

2. " I depend upon other people even for small needs...."

Important Remedy : Sang.

Let us think about this Rubric Today : 12

DELUSION, disorder objects appear in,

Patient Versions :

1. "Doctor….I think, there is a gap between what I say and what you understand…..!"

2. "Sir….I am not definite about the treatments taken by me….Whether…it is going in the right direction or not….."

3. " I cannot understand my problem

properly….sir….!"

Remedies : glon, op.

Note : We cannot confuse this rubric with

"Groping as if in the dark"

Let us think about this Rubric Today : 13

'DELUSIONS - sheep - driving'.

This rubric is very important to understand the full picture of Aconite.

'sheep' means "nothing serious".

Sheep - A meek unimaginative and easily lead animal
Driving - Forcing along, riding, pushing briskly sends always with force, tending towards a point.

Inference - The person feels that the job in hand is like a sheep, which can easily be taken care of.

Remedy : Aconite.

Let us Think about this Rubric Today :14

DELUSION, wrong done, wrong he has,

The patient is my friend. He is a Head Master of a High school. Male age 42.

He has more Duty conscious. He wants to do anything better.
 He had Pain in the lumber region. He has been suffering from this pain for so many days.
 The conversation :
 D: What happened to you sir...?

P; " Nothing sir.....I have pain In the hip side of my back. I cannot start my two wheeler. If I kick the kicker, the pain will become heavy...."
 D: "For how many days do you have this

pain....?"

 P: " May be about more than fifteen days.....":

D: " What did you do for this...."
P : 'Nothing....I that It will be cured as itself...But yesterday when I lay down...severe pain....very less sleep....every night I am not sleeping well due to this pain"

D: "Any thing happened before 15 days....."

P: "......mmm......Sir.......nearly 20 days back, I want to dispose all old news papers, old test papers in my school. (as he is the Head master) So I asked a old paper vendor to collect them. He weighed all that old papers and told that costs of nearly one thousand.....but then he had no such large amount.... So I permitted him to collect all the papers and asked him to pay the next day.. He agreed and went along with all the old papers…..But he did not turn even today….that papers are not mine….It was the property of the school, government….that old paper vendor cheated me…..I did mistake and made a loss to the school….."

D: "Ok…don't worry about that silly persons…You did not do that purposefully …don't worry….anything else do you want to say….?

P:"Nothing…..Sir..

The remedy : HELLIBOURS NIGER.

was given in 30c potency and PL for 15 days.. hibiscus::hibiscus: Very next day when I saw him he told that last night he had slept well…When he started his two wheeler that pain was less…not much….Within few days he was normal free from all pains.
Rubrics Taken :

ANGER, interruption, form,
INDIFFERENCE,   suffering, to
DELUSION, wrong done wrong he has,
Disturbed, averse to being.
DELUSION, crime committed a crime,
he had.

Let us think about this Rubric Today :15

1. Delusion, hands bound with chains,

2. Delusion, hens bound with chains.

 1. Delusion, hands bounded with chains,

Implies he has not able to do anything as he wish for a given situation.
The reason may be either physical of some morality (due to some moral values, he has

For eg:

Nowadays school teachers are not allowed to give punishment (as per Govt. Law) to students for any reasons though the teachers are well wishes of the students. So a dedicated school teacher may feel that his hand is bound with chain, whenever, a student is misbehaving or not studying well, etc.,

We also comparatively study about the Rubric: *Delusion, seized as if,*

In broad manner The Rubric ,
Delusion, Possessed
– is also be considered.

Hyos. Is common to all the above three rubrics.

2. The another beautiful rubric is

Delusion hens bound with chains,
    Here, hen is a harmless domestic birds, in which no need to protect them by bounding them with a heavy chain, just a bamboo basket can do the work.

It is like *"Using Axe for plucking flowers"*

So this is the condition (feelings) for a Timidly person. Even a word can control them not to do some things. For them no need of any heavy protection, etc.,

<u>*Let us think about this Rubric Today :16*</u>

DELUSION, body parts, brown is

Only Remedy : bell

Patient's Versions :

Sir, see...my hair is getting fading..

Due to this hot son, my body getting dim...

Let us think about this Rubric Today : 17

Delusion, servants, must get rid of

Only remedy : fl-ac.

Here Servants are persons who are appointed by us to help.

But the patient is in thought of that they must be send out...as they feel that the servants are unwanted burdens, though they are useful.

Versions:

"Sir...I don't want continue this spectacles. Please give me medicine to improve my vision, so as to read without this spectacles. I feel very uneasy.

Let us think about this Rubric Today : 18

Delusion, sward is hanging over head

Only remedy : am.m.

Versions

"Dr... disease that I have is very dangerous. At any time it will kill me..."

"Sir.. My body condition is not so good, I will fall into the bed at any time.."

Let us think about this Rubric Today : 19

FILLS, Pockets with anything,

The Only Remedy : Stramonium.

Directly speaking it is a Childish behavior.

But if we think in metamorphic way, we can use it in various situations, which are applied to all.

1. He is an Impulsive. He buys everything that he sees, if it is useful, necessary or not.

2. If he visits a book exhibition, He buy so many books, whether if he has time to read or not.

3. He added himself into various Whatsapp, Telegram, Face book groups. Whenever he see a invite link.

4. He accepts every treatment – therapy , advised by his friends and relatives of anybody.

5. Some of Kleptomaniacs persons also considered in this platform.

____

Let us think about this Rubric Today : 20

FRIGHTENED, easily by pains from

Only Remedy : Sulpher

- ❖ He does not allow any surgery, even simple in his body.
- ❖ He will not undertake any responsibilities, because of this fear (Pain = "Care", "Responsibility")

Patient versions :

- ➢ "I came to Homoeopathy, for that reason Allopath put Injections…"

➢ "I am frightened about the care and responsibilities of the new positions, if I promoted..

Let us Think about this Rubric Today : 21

Fear, Paralysis of

A female of age 68 Unmarried.

She was a retired mid-day-meals coordinator. She is doing social service for socially downtrodden people. She has a bicycle to travel in the local to do services.

She has sever pain in the both legs below the knee. Swelling in the both legs. She had suffered nearly one year.

As soon as she entered into my chamber she removed his 'sari" up to her knee and said, "From the toe to knee server pain doctor... see it has swelling.....I have taken so many treatments..But no use...I have taken treatment from Dr.....(well-known Allopath in our home town)....and Dr.......(A popular Ortho.). But no relief."

"I am getting fear about this pain, where I have been unable to walk...."

"Dr...... If I use bicycle for long time......the pain will increase..

" I thought about eye bewitched. So I went to nearby Temple to meet the priest. He gave me a scared thread to wear...."

" Sir(My old patient) already told me that your are giving treatment...But Where is time…?..One after another so many works….”I am doing all the works with this pain….”

"By the by…Sir….12th of this month I am going to Thirupathi. I have an offer to walk from Thirupathi to Thirumala….I once prayed to Lord. So please Dr……cure me before 12th of this month……”

This is her narration. I did not speak even a single work to that patient.

I Took following Rubrics :

1. Business talks of,

2. Naked wants to be,

3. Boaster braggart,

4. Anxiety, pains about,

5. Superstitious,

6. Carried Desire to be, fast

7. Fear, Paralysis of

Bellodona in 30c potency and SL for 15 days were given.

After few days her pain completely gone. Swelling reduced. As she planned, she went Thirumala by walk from down to up (nearly 13 km. in mountain steps), without any relapse of pain!.

Let us think about this Rubric Today : 22

GIFTS, to his wife or son, husband making no.

Only Remedy : Lach

It is an interesting Rubric.

Though wife or son are most lovable by an husband, he does not give any gift to them.

So we may take him as a "Miser" or Niggard Person.

<u>*Let us think about this Rubric Today : 23*</u>

HOUSEKEEPING, Women inapt for,

Important Remedies : LYC, nux.v, sil, sulph.

This is an interesting Rubric, for which, generally women are capable of housekeeping.

But she is a "Modern Woman" who does not know housekeeping.

<u>Let us think about this Rubric Today: 24</u>

INDEPENDENT, Cannot be,

Since This Rubric is self explanatory, I give a case to get better understanding…

Remedies : calc., kiss, nat-m

A case :

Once a school going boy, age 14, come to me for treatment of his complaints.

As I knew his family already and they were living nearby my house,
he asked me, "Sir, my mother asked you give me medicines…."

I asked, "What is your complaints…..?"

He replied, "I have digestion problems, immediately after the food I have to go to toilet...my mother told to say this and to asked to get medicines from you sir...."

I again asked, "Any other complaints....?"

He replied, " My mother told that my stomach is bulged....for that she told to get medicines form you....."

He repeatedly said, "My mother asked this...that..etc.", to get medicines for him form me...

So I took the entry rubric : Independent, cannot be,

He is obstinate. Since he has been known for me for the past few years,

I took the rubric : Obstinate – children, fat, inclined to grow..

I prescribed : Calc. Carb. 200 c one dose.

It worked beautifully, His complaints disappeared within few days (His Mother told me..!).

Now he is studying Engineering in a reputed college, staying at Hostel..!

Let us think about this Rubric Today :25

LONGING, sun shine, light and society

- He is always Happy and Enthusiastic. He has an immense like in something   (as a person, condition, or influence) that radiates warmth, cheer, or happiness.

The Following Patient versions help you to get Better Understanding.

1. " Sir, I don't to be alone. Always I want to go parties, marriage functions etc.,

2. "For how many days I will be in bed…? There is no enjoyment…!"

3. "I want go for a tour….and see some places…..But can't.."

4. "I want to see people…..fresh air to breath….!"

✚ A case:

✚ Once a widow patient of age around 65 was consulted me for severe knee pain in both knees for the past six months.

She lost her husband in a massive attack suddenly, a year before. As a member of an Orthodox Hindu family, she was not allowed to go out side of her home. She has feeling of being neglected.

She wished to go to any functions,
like marriage along with her family
members, even though she couldn't
walk properly. For that she asked
 pain killers for a temprarory relief.

Taking the rubrics :
Company desire for amel, In company
Longing, sunshine

I prescribed Stromonium 6.

After a few days, she became normal,
relieved from her pain.

Let us think about this Rubric Today : 26

Let us think about the Rubrics which are just Opposite to each other

PUNCTUALITY, always on time,

- arg-n, aur-ars, kali-n

LATE, Always,

- calc, cand-a, plat, puls, sil.

(Meaning is self explained)

Let us think about this Rubric Today : 27

SADNESS, Marasmus in.

Only Remedy : ABROT.

Patient Versions :

 "Sir,...I feel very sad, that my body is going to weak day by day...."

This Rubric may be compared with "Delusion thin is getting"

INDEX

Sl. No	Topic	Page No.
1	**P**reface	3
2	**Let us think about this Rubrics Today**	5
3	MIND, Anger, Interruption from	12
4	MIND, Anger, Understood when not	10
5	MIND, Answers, hardly	6
6	MIND, Bending, forward agg.	19
7	MIND, Business, incapacity of	21
8	MIND, Busy, Weak, busy and	16
9	MIND, Carries things to and again back	26
10	MIND, Curious, training of the physician, wants to know the	24
11	MIND, Delusions, blood is not circulates well	33
12	MIND, Delusions, body parts, brown is	44
13	MIND, Delusions, disorder objects appear in	35
14	MIND, Delusions, hands bound with chains,	41
15	MIND, Delusions, hens bound with chains	41
16	MIND, Delusions, Paralyzed being, (he is)	34

17	MIND, Delusions, servants, must get rid of	45
18	MIND, Delusions, sheep, driving	36
19	MIND, Delusions, sward is hanging over head	46
20	MIND, Delusions, wrong done, wrong he has	37
21	MIND, Disturbed, averse to being	29
22	MIND, Fear, paralysis of	51
23	MIND, Fills, pockets with anything,	47
24	MIND, Frightened, easily by pain from	49
25	MIND, Gifts, to his wife of son, husband making no	55
26	MIND, Housekeeping, women inapt for,	56
27	MIND, Independent, cannot be,	57
28	MIND, Late, always	63
29	MIND, Longing, sunshine, light and society	60
30	MIND, Punctuality, always on time	63
31	MIND, Sadness, Marasums in	64